What is Youth?
A Fool's Guide to Staying Young in 5 Easy Steps
by Susana McGuire Jewell

Published by Susana McGuire Jewell

PO Box 2273
Monterey, CA 93942

Find us on the Web at:

www.whatisyouth.com
or www.deliciousyoga.net

Copyright © 2014 by Susana McGuire Jewell
Cover & Interior design: McGuire Communication

Notice of Rights: All rights reserved. No part of this book may be reproduced or transmitted in any form by any means, electronic, mechanical, photocopying, recording, or otherwise, without the prior written permission of the publisher.

For information on getting permission for reprints and excerpts, contact: Email: mcguirecommunication@yahoo.com

Susana McGuire Jewell does not claim to practice medicine, prescribe for or diagnose disease; does not hold out, state, indicate, advertise or imply that she is a licensed physician. The materials and content contained in this book are for general education only and are not intended to be a substitute for professional medical advice, diagnosis or treatment. Users of this book should not rely exclusively on information provided in this book for their own health needs. All specific medical questions should be presented to your own health care provider.

TABLE OF CONTENTS

INTRODUCTION

This book is about an investigation to turning back the clock.

Personally, I was just a moderately athletic kid, and absolutely hated gym class. I wasn't always thin, wasn't always strong. And I seemed to have every illness. I spent a lot of time drawing and listening to music.

In the early 80's while attending art school, I lived with dancers in a cockroach infested tenement in Manhattan. While I studied figure drawing, color, line and sculpture, they would dance all day. One of them for the American Ballet Theater.

At night, they washed their leotards in the bathtub and went out and danced again all the next day. The books on their shelves were *Diet for a Small Planet* by Frances Moore Lappé, *Back to Eden* by Jethro Kloss, etc.

I was introduced to massage, herbs, millet, gravity boots, acupressure, and a health club called Jack LaLanne where I learned to lift weights and dance. I became a runner, running around the Central Park Reservoir... and my body literally sang with freedom.

Long story short, I caught the fitness/health bug although my diet still contained mostly 90% sugar.

I got stronger, walking around the city got a lot easier, and I liked what I saw in the mirror.

At 50+ now I can say my workouts have gone up and down in intensity, and have included some short periods in-between when I was quite inactive.

But what has forged the steely resolve I have now? Seeing the precious people in my family slowly decompose and become the living dead from sedentariness, sugar, fat and white flour - lack of nutrients; poor lifestyle choices. They are in heaven now, and I became a personal trainer. If I can save anyone from going down the road to the living dead, I've done my job. As the life force drained out of them all, the question that started to haunt me is... ***WHAT IS YOUTH?***

WHAT IS YOUTH?

The dictionary says:

- *the state or quality of being young*
  esp. as associated with vigor, freshness or immaturity

How does vigor & freshness get lost, and why does immaturity have a bad name... is it too **foolish**?

I'll go on to say that youth may just be ZEST.

Associated with courage, Zest is defined as living life with a sense of excitement, anticipation, and energy. Approaching life as an adventure. Fools rush in where angels, or the middle aged, fear to tread.

Those who have Zest exude excitement and energy while living life. The concept of zest involves performing tasks wholeheartedly, while also being adventurous, vivacious and energetic.
Va Va VOOOM!

Where does this all go to when the years fly by?

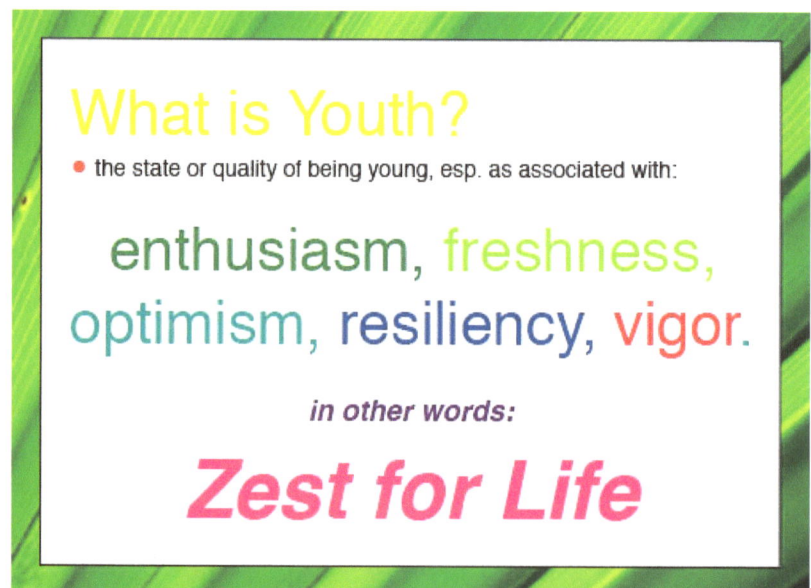

One thing led to another and I wondered -

WHAT ARE OUR BODIES FOR?

"Your body belongs to your ancestors, your parents, and future generations, and it also belongs to society and all other living beings. All of them have come together to bring about the presence of this body. Keeping your body healthy is an expression of gratitude to the whole cosmos — the trees, the clouds, everything."

— Thich Nhat Hanh, "Touching Peace"

Apparently it's our duty to take care of this miracle flesh suit were are inside of. And our deepest responsibility.

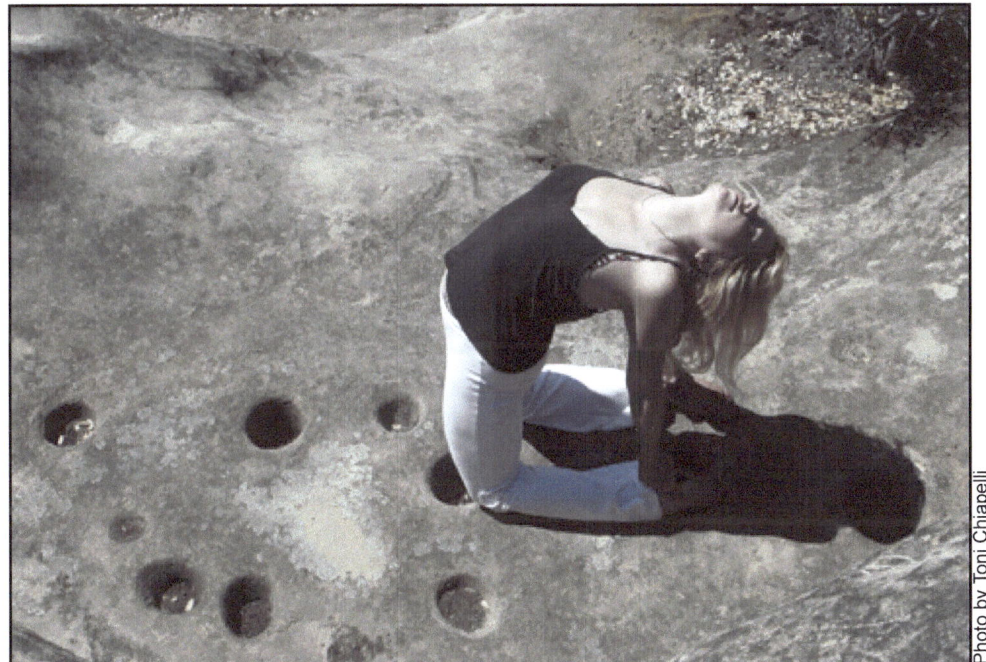

Susana in Ustransa at Los Padres National Forest CA

I teach Hatha Yoga and Power Yoga. Hatha Yoga is a type of yoga that acknowledges the body's presence to such a degree that while involved in the practice of this yoga (and it is a practice), enlightenment can be obtained **through** the body – not in spite of it.

We have a body. It is our vehicle. And through it, we may know our divinity.

LIFE EXPECTANCY

So, life is a very interesting experience, and here we are in it. Every person who has ever lived on this planet has had the same experience - being alive in a human body.

The thing that is interesting now - what is different from the past - is the huge gain in life expectancy.

My grandmother (who lived to be 87), often told the story of an old lady in her neighborhood. The woman sat on her porch wrapped in a shawl rocking in a chair. Gramma (as a young child) with her friends would scurry about to sneak peaks at her and whisper... "She's sooo old... she's half a hundred!" (50.) My grandmother said she never expected to live as long as she did.

Now living until 100 years old is becoming common. Some experts predict age 120 will be common with children born today. What will happen when you and I are in our 90's? Maybe it's time to think ahead.

As John Mellencamp said, "Oh yeah – life goes on long after the thrill of living is gone." When the song came out and I was young, I had no idea what he meant. Now I do.

At 51 right now I consider myself a Senior In Training.

Face it. You may be around for a lot longer than you were planning. My advice is to plan ahead. Think about it – you may have to go the distance.

I have personally seen the grisly result of life being extended for the completely lifeless in nursing homes. How does that happen? My personal feeling is that it happens very very gradually... so slow that the loss of vitality, strength and range of motion is hard to pinpoint.

You can take action *now* to literally build a body that will be fun to be inside of for many years to come. The prescription is exercise. Movement that is fun, daily, and includes a diet that supports the optimal functioning of this glorious machine you are driving.

THE 5 STEPS

I have found these 5 steps to be very effective through 11 years of teaching hundreds upon hundreds of folks from all walks of life; all sizes, all ability levels and all ages.

I even teach a class I call Stretch Therapy for seniors and folks with movement disabilities.

And I make them all...

1. SIT ON THE FLOOR

What??????? Are you nuts? I haven't sat on the floor since I've was a child!

Immature? Foolish?

....oh.... children sit on the floor. Always.

Do you know what sitting in a chair or on a couch does to your body for years? Your hip flexors become chronically tightened, pulling your back into a slump, and your buttocks turn soft. The abdominals atrophy. All this can lead to lower back pain and a myriad of more problems.

Sitting up tall on the floor can get rid of that brain fog, and waken up your mind and spirit as all your organs are right where they are intended to be.

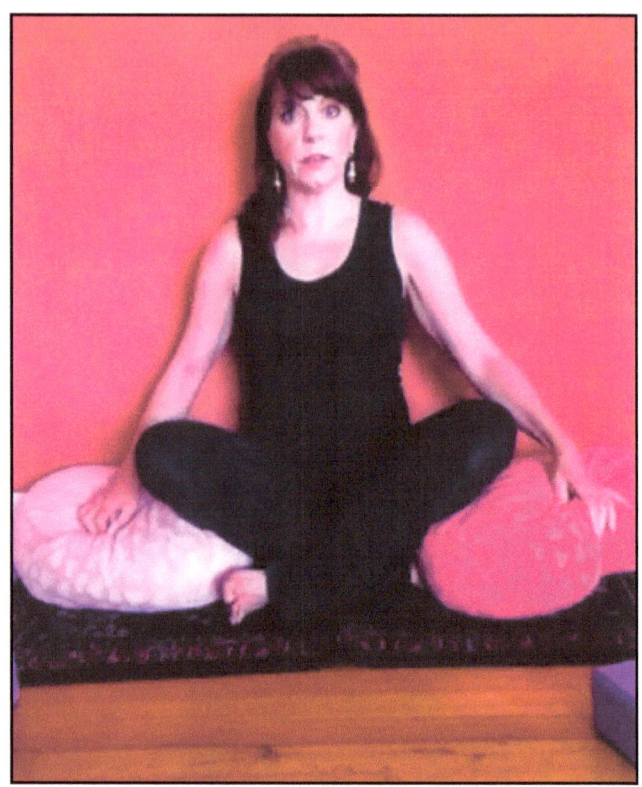

YOUR HOMEWORK:

Figure 1 **Seated on Pillow** (with pillows under knees if needed)

Sit in the floor for all or part of one television show.

If you don't watch TV or your computer, do it for part of a conversation with a friend.

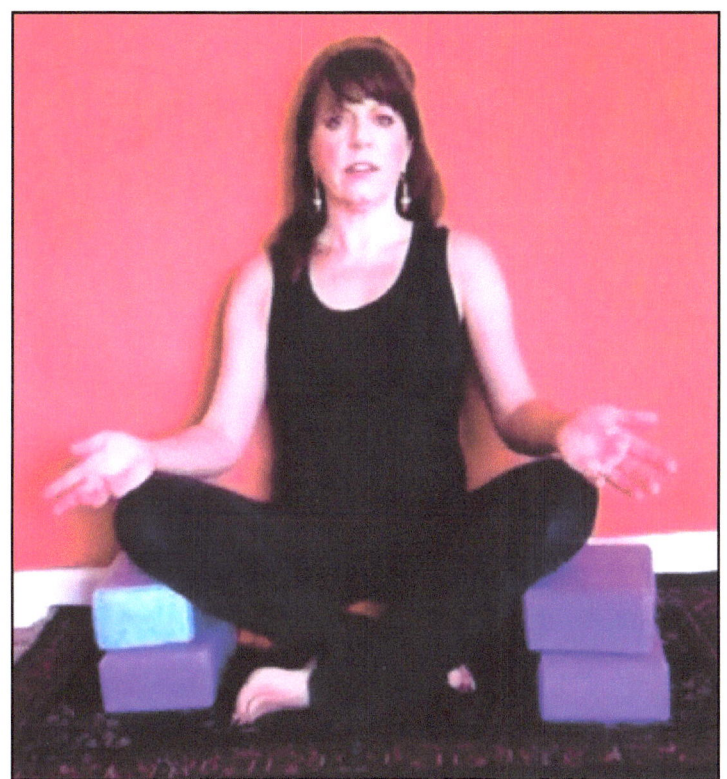

Figure 2 **SEATED ON A PILLOW** (with blocks under knees if needed)

If it's hard to sit up tall, you can sit cross legged on a pillow with your back against a wall, with blocks under your knees.

Do either of these once a day for a small amount of time building to 20 minutes per day.

Your posture will improve and your hips will get more flexible, improving your lower back.

2. STRETCH DAILY

Flexibility is a key component of physical fitness.

Also, age is often associated with a sedentary lifestyle. And the older we are, the tighter we get.

Did you know that flexibility is the range of motion around your joints, and that you can change that?

...And any progress you may make today in increasing that range of motion is actually lost tomorrow if you don't stretch again.

Wow. Sounds like work. But with the simple stretches I'm going to show you, it is quick, doable, and feels delicious.

Do these stretches once or twice a day, upon rising or before bed; or at the very least, several times a week.

You can be on the floor, or actually do these in bed.

Hold each stretch for a few moments while breathing deeply. The breathing facilitates the stretch. Inhale, exhale.

Easing into at least 30 seconds for each stretch to one minute. Stretching has to feel good to be affective.

Make it feel good - that's your job.

How? Relax your spine into the floor or bed, CLOSE YOUR EYES, and keep breathing deeply.

Do not force. Let gravity do the work. Stretching takes time. Put the time in and your body will be in appreciation.

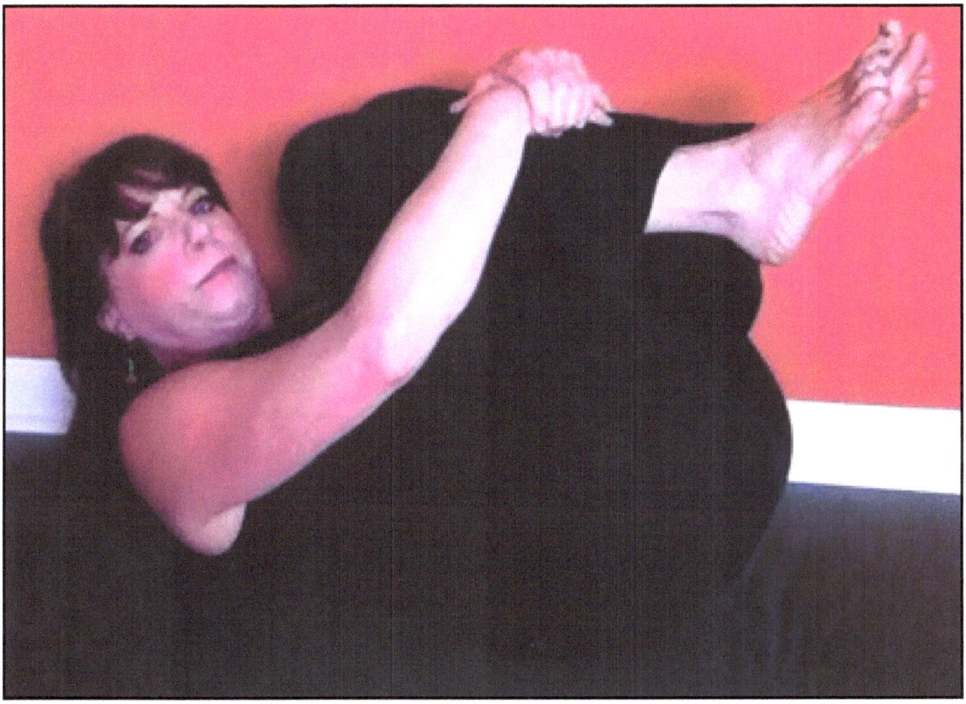

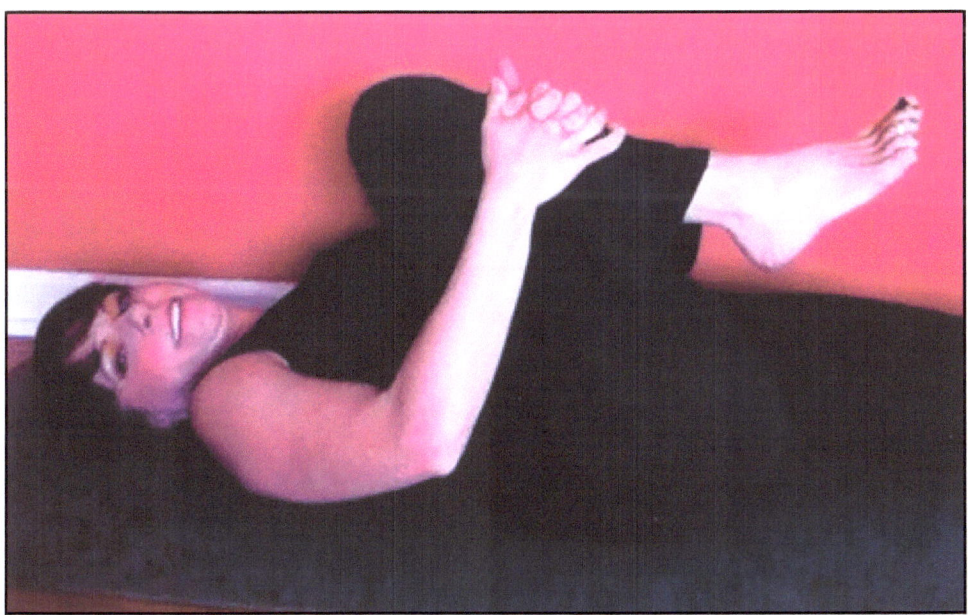

Figure 3 **KNEES TO CHEST SQUEEZE**. Stretches the Erector Spinae, the spinal stabilizer muscles.

Figure 4 **ONE KNEE TO CHEST**, with other leg straight. Stretches the Psoas muscle (the hip flexor) and releases the lower back.

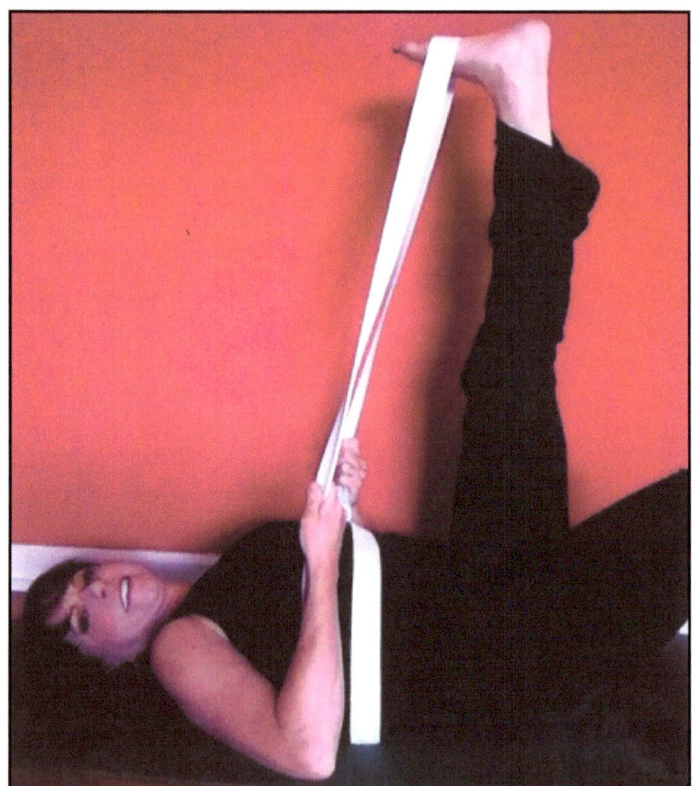

Figure 5 **ONE LEG IN A STRAP**. Stretches the Hamstring muscle (back of the thigh). You can use a soft bathrobe tie or martial art belt.

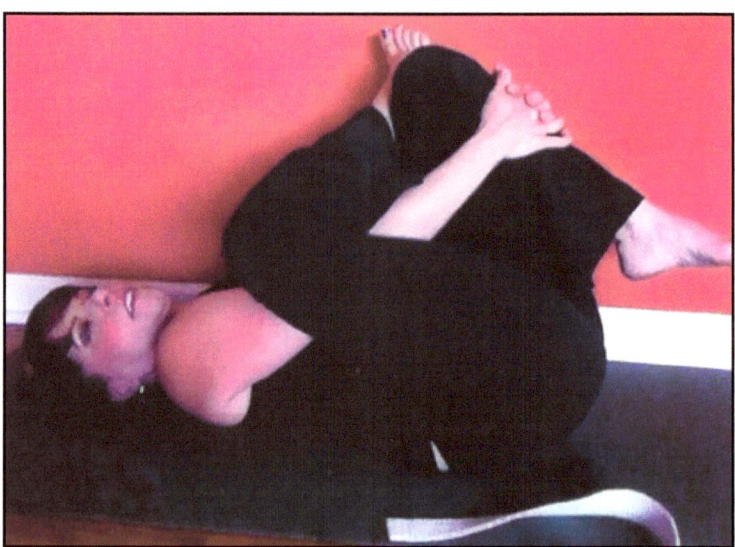

Figure 6 **FIGURE 4 STRETCH**. Make a figure four by putting your ankle on the opposite knee, and threading your hands through your legs. Stretches the Periformis which may bring relief to sciatica.

3. INVERSION

Did you ever see a kid not want to be upside down?

Summersaults, kickstands, hanging upside down on playground equipment - that's fun for a kid!

Silly foolish and young.

Growning brains need plenty of oxygen. Inversions get freshly oxygenated blood to the brain. That doesn't change when we get older.

Regular inversion, experts say, improves your concentration, memory, observation and clarity of thought. And the brain operates 14% more accurately when your body is in an inverted or inclined plane.

Put simply, turning your world upside down makes your brain better.

And it calms the mind.

Another thing to do in bed!

Any inversion should be avoided if you have serious eye problems such as glaucoma, or unchecked high blood pressure.

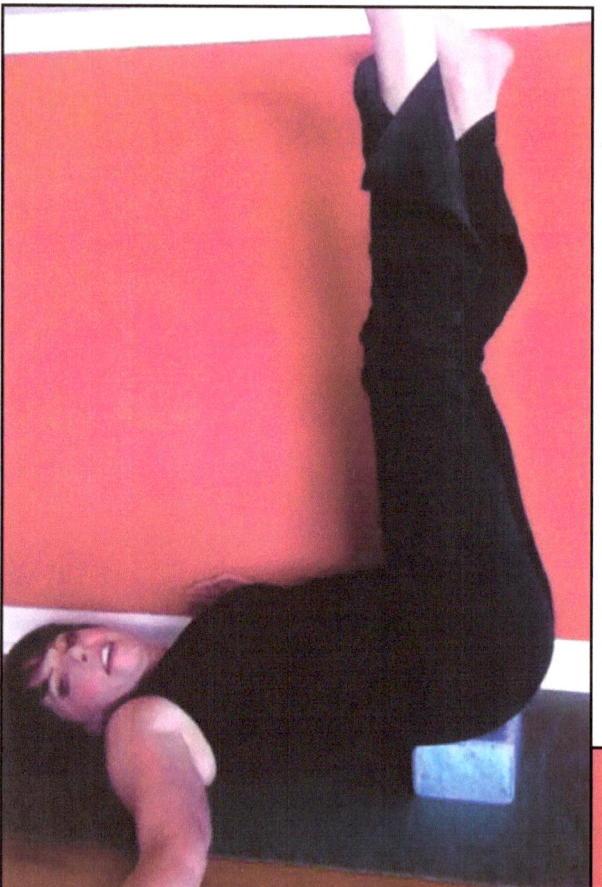

Figure 7
INVERSION WITH A BLOCK
(or ball or pillow)

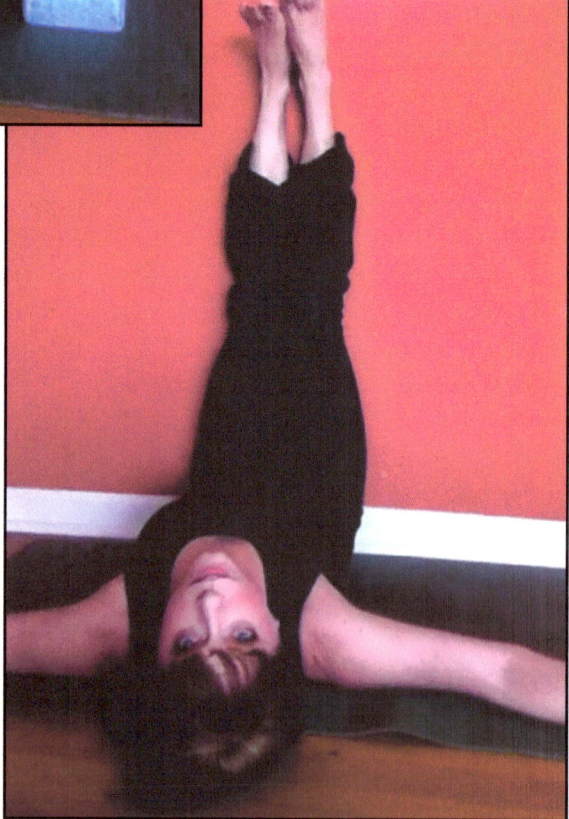

Fig 8
LEGS UP THE WALL
(can be done on your bed)

4. EAT A CLEAN DIET

What's a clean diet? Fruits, vegetables, whole grains, and lean proteins. Heard that before? Why is it hard? Perhaps convenience, perhaps no one around you is eating this way - peer pressure. I remember my family literally laughing at my foolish diet.

Did you know this diet is quite cost effective?

You can just cut up fruits and vegetables, add a slice of whole grain bread, some raw nuts and take it to work to snack on. But why do that?

Here's Your Motivation:
A study of 65,226 men and women indicated the more fruit and vegetables people ate, the less likely they were to die – at any age.

Immortality at last.

Or at least mobility and *Zest* as life goes on and on past 90.

So what's the right amount?

Seven-A-Day Fruit and Veg 'Saves Lives'
By Pippa Stephens, Health reporter, BBC News

Eating seven or more portions of fruit and vegetables a day is healthier than the minimum five currently recommended and would prolong lives, experts say.

Seven a day cut the risk of dying from cancer and heart disease.

"The clear message here is that the more fruit and vegetables you eat, the less likely you are to die at any age"

Dr Oyinola Oyebode
Department of Epidemiology and Public Health, UCL

One Way To Get Your 7 is Green Smoothies

Why? Nutrition in, garbage out. (Colon cleanse.) I do this several times per week and my energy has completely turned around.

I start with:
Apple (cored), carrot, celery + tops (or not)
or peaches or whatever is in season
or I get blueberries or strawberries and freeze them myself on a cookie sheet, then store in ziplock bags.

Then add:
Kale, spinach or romaine
Add about 2 cups of water. Blend in blender for a good minute. You want the end result to be totally liquid. The more organic, the better. That's it!

Or you also add one or more of the following:
Ice
A couple of dates, or other dried fruit, or stevia for sweetness
peeled de-seeded cucumber
avocado or banana for thickness and even more nutrients
garlic, and/or hunk of peeled ginger
protein powder

Anything goes
and your energy level will
thank you.

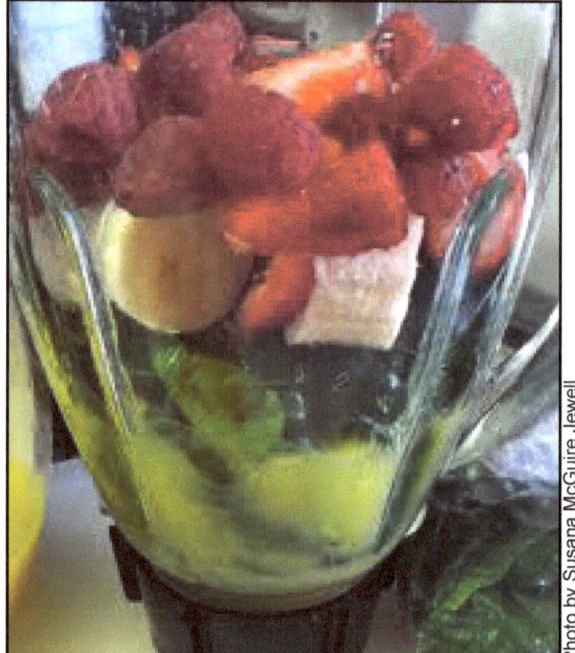

5. APPRECIATION

Appreciate what? All I see is what I don't have and what I need. I see what others have that I don't.

But look deeper. Close your eyes and take a deeeep breath. You can breathe. You can hear. You can see. You can feel.

Start with something very small - if you are in your home, find something in the room that makes you happy. Do you have a nice memory with that object? Was it a gift?

If you are in your bed - is it soft? Are the sheets cool on your skin? Your pillow fluffy?

This might seem foolish. How are we supposed to get ahead in the rat race doing this?

Well, one thought of appreciation (just one)... if you hold onto it for a few moments will grow bigger and latch onto another thought like it.

Like attracts like.

Then another happy thought gets added to the chain. Then another. Soon your appreciation grows larger and larger. So what? Big deal?

The big deal is that those big appreciative thoughts will attract *like* events to your world. Good things start with good thoughts. And good thoughts start with just one thought.

For an added bonus, the body & mind responds to appreciation (or gratitude), joy, smiling, and the relaxation that follows by releasing healthy hormones to every cell.

So use your mind to change your world.

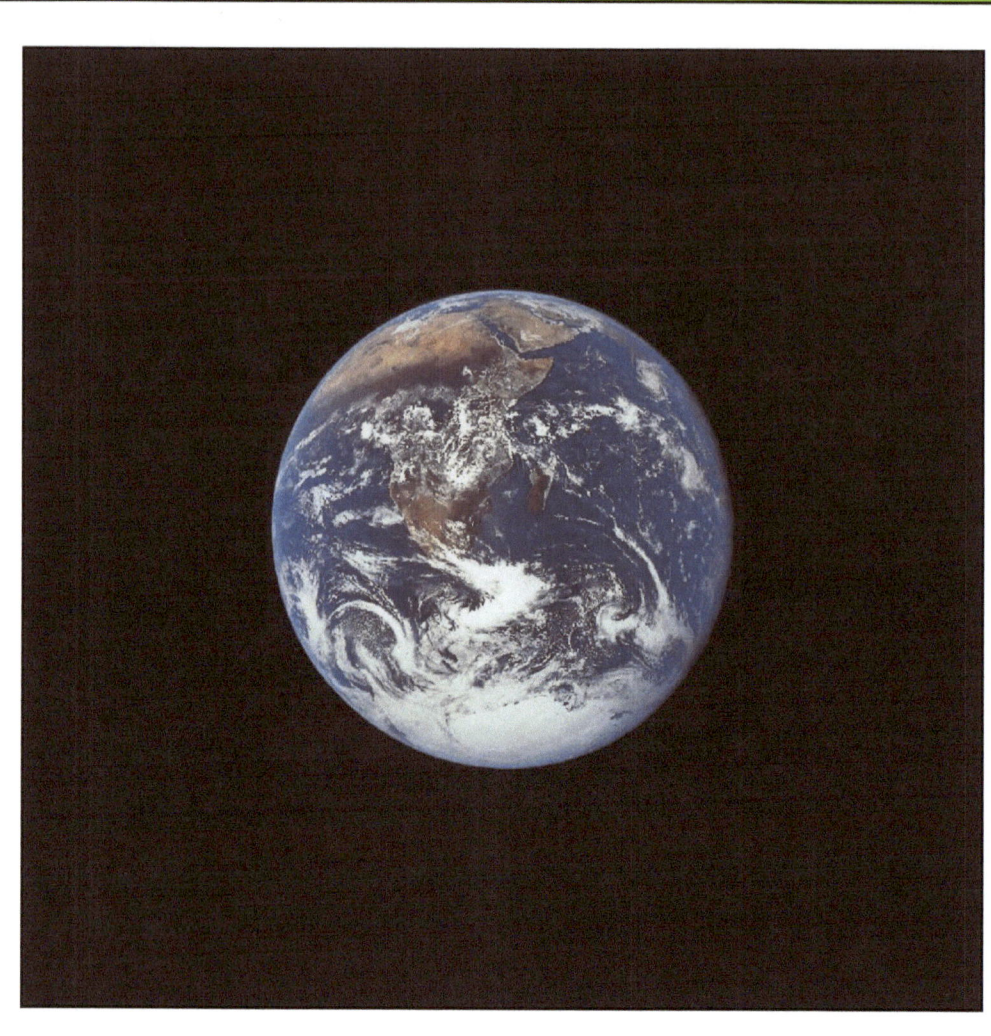

IN CONCLUSION

The Five Foolish Steps:

1. Sit On The Floor
2. Stretch Daily
3. Inversion
4. Clean Diet
5. Appreciate

Do these daily and watch the pleasant changes.

Email me with your results - I'd love to hear about it.

susana.mcguire@gmail.com

I also provide webinars and workshops to delve deeper into each five Zesty steps above as well as more in-depth stretching, yoga and exercise.

In addition, there are upcoming books, workshops and tutorials on more Stay Young Strategies, fitness and diet.

Send me an email to be updated on the dates. And please forward this information to loved ones of yours who could use a bit of Zest.

Stay young, my friend.

~Susana

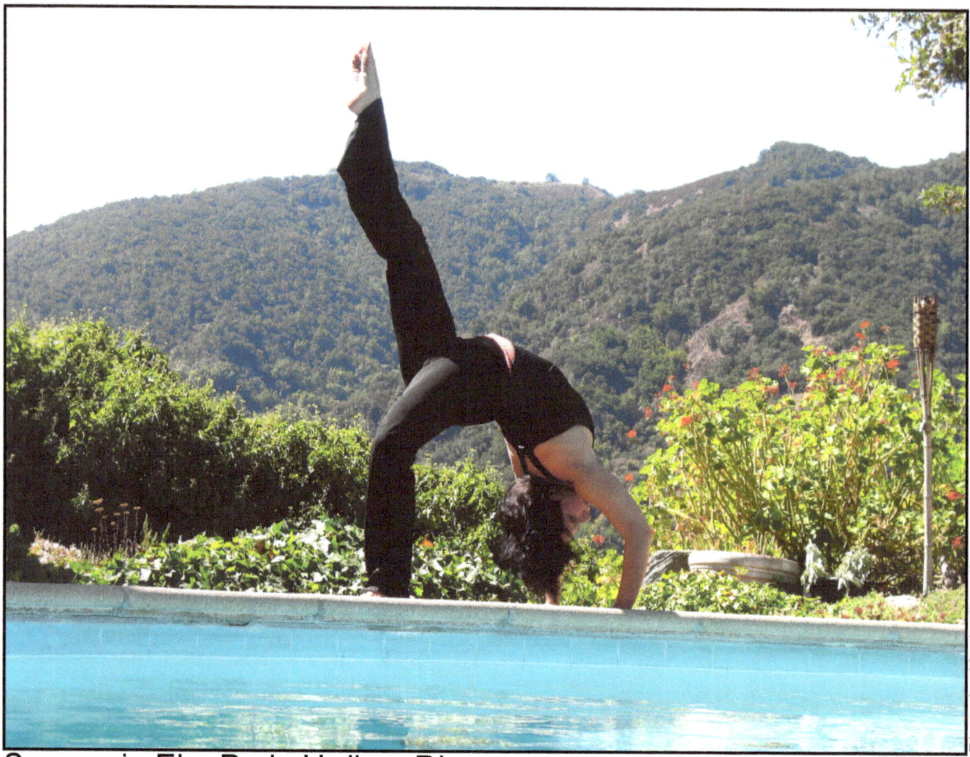

Susana in Eka Pada Urdhva Dhanurasana

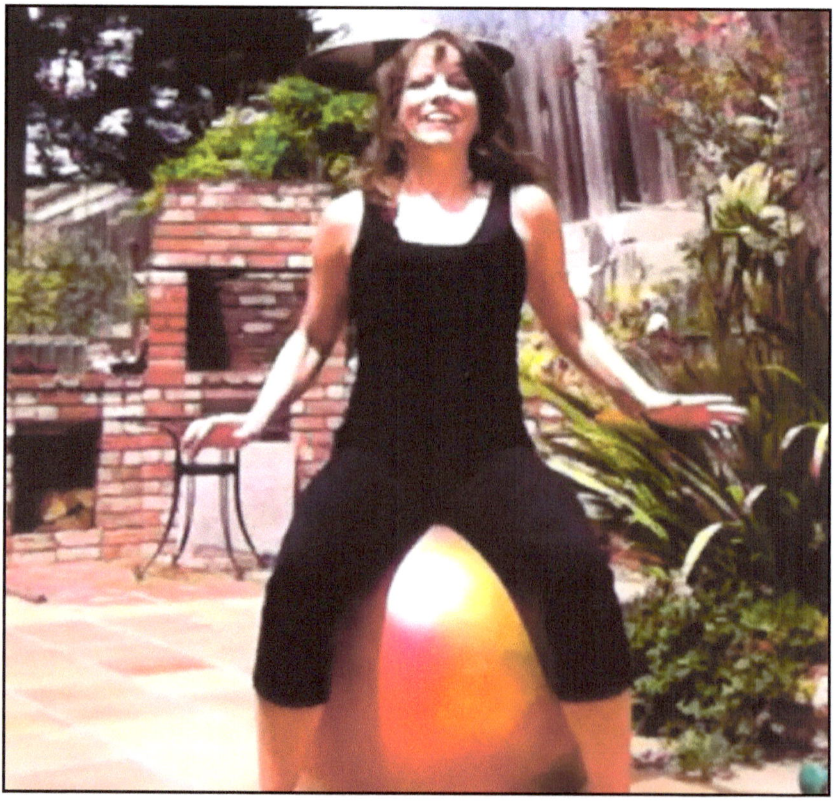

About Susana

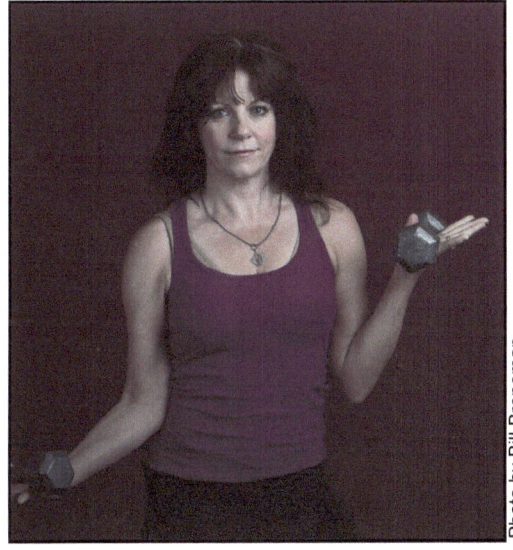

Photo by Bill Breneman

Susana McGuire Jewell is a business owner, artist, designer, singer and fitness expert.

At 50+, Susana helps people everyday to get stronger, more fit and more flexible - and live more in this moment right now.

Her favorite pastimes are cooking healthy food, entertaining, riding her bike along the Monterey Bay, hanging out with her husband, friends and cats.

She is a graduate of Parsons School of Design in Manhattan and holds a B.F.A. in Communication Design.

Susana is certified by the Aerobics and Fitness Association of America (AFAA) as a Personal Trainer.

She is also a Certified Yoga Instructor, and has over 11 years of experience teaching weekly classes in hatha yoga, power yoga Pilates, aerobics and weight training.

susana.mcguire@gmail.com
www.whatisyouth.com
www.deliciousyoga.net
www.susanamcguire.com

Notes

Notes

Notes

www.ingramcontent.com/pod-product-compliance
Lightning Source LLC
Chambersburg PA
CBHW050933290526
45792CB00002B/1002